Leptin Resistance Diet

A Beginner's 3-Step Plan to Managing Leptin Resistance Through Diet, with Sample Recipes and a 7-Day Meal Plan

mf

copyright © 2022 Brandon Gilta

All rights reserved No part of this book may be reproduced, or stored in a retrieval system, or transmitted in any form or by any means, electronic, mechanical, photocopying, recording, or otherwise, without express written permission of the publisher.

Disclaimer

By reading this disclaimer, you are accepting the terms of the disclaimer in full. If you disagree with this disclaimer, please do not read the guide.

All of the content within this guide is provided for informational and educational purposes only, and should not be accepted as independent medical or other professional advice. The author is not a doctor, physician, nurse, mental health provider, or registered nutritionist/dietician. Therefore, using and reading this guide does not establish any form of a physician-patient relationship.

Always consult with a physician or another qualified health provider with any issues or questions you might have regarding any sort of medical condition. Do not ever disregard any qualified professional medical advice or delay seeking that advice because of anything you have read in this guide. The information in this guide is not intended to be any sort of medical advice and should not be used in lieu of any medical advice by a licensed and qualified medical professional.

The information in this guide has been compiled from a variety of known sources. However, the author cannot attest to or guarantee the accuracy of each source and thus should not be held liable for any errors or omissions.

You acknowledge that the publisher of this guide will not be held liable for any loss or damage of any kind incurred as a result of this guide or the reliance on any information provided within this guide. You acknowledge and agree that you assume all risk and responsibility for any action you undertake in response to the information in this guide.

Using this guide does not guarantee any particular result (e.g., weight loss or a cure). By reading this guide, you acknowledge that there are no guarantees to any specific outcome or results you can expect.

All product names, diet plans, or names used in this guide are for identification purposes only and are the property of their respective owners. The use of these names does not imply endorsement. All other trademarks cited herein are the property of their respective owners.

Where applicable, this guide is not intended to be a substitute for the original work of this diet plan and is, at most, a supplement to the original work for this diet plan and never a direct substitute. This guide is a personal expression of the facts of that diet plan.

Where applicable, persons shown in the cover images are stock photography models and the publisher has obtained the rights to use the images through license agreements with third-party stock image companies.

Table of Contents

Introduction   7
All About Leptin   10
   Can leptin levels be controlled?   11
   What causes leptin resistance?   13
   Symptoms of leptin resistance   14
   How is leptin resistance diagnosed?   15
Focusing on Leptin Receptor Deficiency   17
   Understanding Leptin Receptors   17
   How Is Leptin Resistance Treated?   21
Managing Leptin Resistance through Diet   24
   Principles of the Leptin Diet   24
   Benefits of The Leptin Diet   26
   Disadvantages of the Leptin Diet   28
5 Step-by-Step Guide on How to Get Started with the Leptin Diet   31
   Step 1: Understand the Basics of Leptin   31
   Step 2: Plan Your Meals   32
   Meal Planning Tips   36
   Step 3: Follow Structured Eating Times   37
   Step 4: Incorporate Regular Exercise   39
   Step 5: Monitor Your Progress   41
   Foods to Eat   46
   Tips on How to Shop for Leptin Sensitivity-Boosting Foods   50
   Foods to Avoid   51
Meal Plans to Add to Your Leptin-Resistance Diet   56
   A 7-Day Meal Plan   58
Sample Recipes   59
   Salmon with Sweet Potato and Kale   60
   No-Fuss Tuna Casserole   61

Pecan and Maple Salmon	62
Velvety Herbed Pumpkin	63
Greek Salad with Arugula	65
Tuna Salad	67
Chicken Breast with Herbs	68
Creamy Low-FODMAP Fish Casserole	69
Green and Berry Smoothie	71
Healthy Green Smoothie	72
Mediterranean Breakfast	73
Carrot Cake Oats	74
Fresh Cucumber Salad	75
Quinoa Lentil Salad	76
Strawberry, Blueberry, and Spinach Salad	78
Conclusion	**79**
FAQs	**83**
Helpful Questions Regarding Leptin Resistance	84
References and Helpful Links	**86**

Introduction

Are you struggling to manage your weight despite following countless diet plans and exercise regimens? You're not alone. Many individuals embark on their weight loss journey with dedication and hope only to find themselves stuck in a frustrating cycle of minimal results. What's often overlooked in these efforts is the role of hormones, specifically leptin—the "satiety hormone"—that plays a crucial role in regulating appetite and metabolism.

Leptin is produced by fat cells and communicates with the brain about the body's energy reserves. When functioning optimally, leptin signals the brain that you're full and have enough energy stored, thereby reducing hunger and promoting calorie burning. However, factors like chronic dieting, overeating, stress, and lack of sleep can disrupt leptin sensitivity, leading to leptin resistance. This condition makes it difficult for the brain to recognize satiety, causing persistent hunger and reduced metabolic rate.

Understanding and managing leptin levels can be a game-changer for those seeking sustainable weight management. The Leptin Management Diet Guide is designed to help you restore leptin sensitivity naturally through targeted dietary strategies and lifestyle modifications. By focusing on balanced nutrition, proper meal timing, and specific foods that enhance leptin function, this guide aims to support long-term health and weight goals.

This guide will also help you with the following:

- Learn more about leptin and leptin resistance
- How leptin resistance is diagnosed
- Leptin resistance symptoms
- Food to eat and avoid
- Managing leptin resistance

Consider a life where you feel genuinely satiated after meals, experience fewer cravings, and see consistent progress towards your weight goals. This is the promise of leptin management. By adhering to the principles outlined in this guide, you'll not only enhance your body's natural regulatory mechanisms but also improve overall well-being. You'll gain insights into making smarter food choices, structuring meals effectively, and adopting habits that promote hormonal balance.

The Leptin Management Diet Guide is more than just a diet plan; it's a comprehensive approach to achieving harmony between your eating habits and your body's needs. It's about fostering a healthier relationship with food and leveraging the power of nutrition to support metabolic functions. As you embark on this journey, remember that small, consistent changes can lead to significant improvements over time. Your commitment to understanding and managing leptin will serve as a foundation for a healthier, more vibrant life.

Ready to take control of your health and unlock the potential of leptin management? Dive into the upcoming chapters to discover practical tips, detailed meal plans, and recipes tailored to enhance leptin sensitivity. Whether you're new to the concept or looking to refine your current approach, the Leptin Management Diet Guide will equip you with the knowledge and tools needed for successful, sustainable weight management.

Stay tuned as we explore the intricacies of leptin, uncover the best foods for leptin regulation, and develop a personalized plan that fits seamlessly into your lifestyle. Let's embark on this transformative journey together, one step at a time.

All About Leptin

Leptin is a hormone crucial for regulating energy intake and expenditure. Secreted by fat cells, its blood levels are proportional to the amount of body fat.

A hormone is a signaling molecule produced by an endocrine gland and released into the bloodstream. Upon release, it binds to specific receptors on target cells, triggering a biological response. Hormones regulate numerous physiological processes, including growth and development, metabolism, reproduction, and mood. Hormonal imbalances can lead to various disorders.

The primary function of leptin is to help maintain a healthy weight by regulating food intake and energy expenditure. High leptin levels signal fullness, reducing food consumption, while low levels induce hunger, increasing food intake. Produced by fat cells, leptin is released into the bloodstream in response to food. It then travels to the brain, binds to receptors, and sends signals that regulate hunger and energy use.

Leptin resistance occurs when the body becomes less responsive to leptin's effects. As a result, the body fails to receive the signal to stop eating, leading to overeating and weight gain. This complex condition is not fully understood but is believed to arise from a combination of genetic and environmental factors.

Can leptin levels be controlled?

Leptin levels can be influenced by various factors, including diet, weight, and exercise. Here are some ways to manage leptin levels effectively:

- *Diet*: Consuming foods that enhance leptin sensitivity, such as those rich in fiber, protein, and healthy fats, can help regulate leptin levels. Some examples include leafy green vegetables, nuts, seeds, lean meats, and avocados. Conversely, avoiding processed foods high in sugar and unhealthy fats is crucial as they can promote leptin resistance. Such harmful foods often include sugary snacks, fast food, and ready-to-eat meals, which, in the long term, can disrupt the body's hormonal balance.
- *Weight Management*: Maintaining a healthy weight is crucial for controlling leptin levels. Excess body fat can lead to elevated leptin levels, which may contribute to leptin resistance over time. Adopting a balanced diet and regular physical activity can aid in

achieving and sustaining a healthy weight. It's also important to monitor caloric intake and ensure you're eating a variety of nutrient-dense foods. Additionally, staying hydrated and getting adequate sleep can further support weight management efforts.

- *Exercise*: Regular physical activity has been shown to increase leptin sensitivity. Engaging in both aerobic exercises (such as running, swimming, or cycling) and strength training can improve overall metabolic health and enhance the body's response to leptin. Aerobic exercises help in burning calories and maintaining cardiovascular health, while strength training builds muscle mass, which can improve metabolic rate. A well-rounded exercise routine should also include flexibility and balance exercises to ensure overall fitness and reduce the risk of injury.

Additionally, getting adequate sleep and managing stress levels can also play a role in regulating leptin levels, as poor sleep and chronic stress have been linked to hormonal imbalances, including leptin resistance. By incorporating these lifestyle changes, individuals can better control their leptin levels and support their overall health.

What causes leptin resistance?

Leptin resistance is a complex condition with no single cause, often resulting from a combination of genetic and environmental factors. Here are some potential causes:

- *Obesity*: One of the most significant risk factors for leptin resistance. Excess body fat can lead to higher levels of leptin, which over time may cause the body to become less responsive to the hormone.
- *Inflammation*: Chronic inflammation has been linked to the development of leptin resistance. Inflammatory markers can interfere with leptin signaling, making it harder for the hormone to regulate appetite and metabolism.
- *Blood Sugar Imbalances*: Conditions like type 2 diabetes, which involve imbalances in blood sugar levels, have been associated with leptin resistance. When blood sugar levels are consistently high, it can affect how the body responds to leptin signals.
- *Certain Medications*: Some medications, such as corticosteroids, can increase the risk of developing leptin resistance. These medications can alter the body's hormonal balance and metabolism, potentially leading to resistance over time.

These are just some of the known causes of leptin resistance, but there may be other contributing factors as well.

Symptoms of leptin resistance

Leptin resistance can manifest through a variety of symptoms, often related to hunger, metabolism, and weight management. Common symptoms include:

- *Persistent Hunger*: Despite consuming adequate calories, individuals with leptin resistance often feel continually hungry. This is because the brain does not receive the signal that the body is full, leading to constant cravings and increased appetite.
- *Difficulty Losing Weight*: People with leptin resistance may find it challenging to lose weight, even with diet and exercise. The body's impaired response to leptin disrupts normal metabolic processes, making weight loss more difficult.
- *Weight Gain*: Weight gain, particularly around the abdomen, is a common symptom. The body's inability to regulate energy intake and expenditure efficiently can lead to an accumulation of fat.
- *Fatigue*: Chronic fatigue and low energy levels are frequently reported. Leptin plays a role in regulating energy balance, and resistance to this hormone can lead to feelings of tiredness and lack of motivation.
- *Increased Fat Storage*: The body may store more fat than usual, especially in the abdominal area. This can contribute to an unhealthy body composition and increase the risk of metabolic disorders.

- ***Poor Metabolic Health***: Individuals may exhibit signs of metabolic syndrome, such as high blood pressure, elevated blood sugar levels, and abnormal cholesterol levels. These conditions are often linked to leptin resistance and increase the risk of cardiovascular disease and type 2 diabetes.
- ***Sleep Disturbances***: Leptin resistance can affect sleep patterns, leading to poor-quality sleep or insomnia. Proper leptin function is crucial for regulating circadian rhythms and overall sleep health.

Recognizing these symptoms is important for identifying leptin resistance early and seeking appropriate medical advice. Addressing lifestyle factors such as diet, exercise, and stress management can help improve leptin sensitivity and overall health.

How is leptin resistance diagnosed?

Diagnosing leptin resistance is complex, as there is no single definitive test. Instead, it is identified through a combination of symptoms, medical history, and various diagnostic tests. Here are some methods commonly used to assess leptin resistance:

- ***Blood Tests***: Blood tests are often performed to measure levels of leptin and other related hormones. Elevated leptin levels in the presence of obesity may indicate leptin resistance.

- ***Imaging Tests***: Imaging techniques such as MRI or CT scans can help identify signs of obesity or other underlying conditions that contribute to leptin resistance. These tests provide detailed images of body fat distribution and can reveal visceral fat, which is closely associated with metabolic disorders.
- ***Genetic Tests***: Genetic testing may be conducted to identify mutations associated with leptin resistance. Certain genetic variations can predispose individuals to this condition, and understanding these genetic factors can aid in forming a comprehensive diagnosis.
- ***Clinical Evaluation***: A thorough clinical evaluation, including a review of the patient's medical history and physical examination, is essential. Healthcare providers look for symptoms such as persistent hunger, difficulty losing weight, and signs of metabolic syndrome.
- ***Metabolic Assessments***: Additional assessments, such as glucose tolerance tests or insulin sensitivity tests, may be used to evaluate overall metabolic health. These tests can provide insights into how the body processes sugar and responds to insulin, which are often linked to leptin resistance.

By combining these diagnostic approaches, healthcare providers can form a more accurate understanding of leptin resistance and develop an appropriate treatment plan tailored to the individual's needs.

Focusing on Leptin Receptor Deficiency

When it comes to leptin resistance, there are different types of deficiencies that can occur. One specific type is known as leptin receptor deficiency, which refers to a lack or dysfunction of the receptors responsible for recognizing and responding to leptin in the body.

Understanding Leptin Receptors

Leptin receptors are found on cells throughout the body, including in the hypothalamus (the part of the brain that regulates appetite and metabolism), adipose tissue, liver, and other organs. These receptors bind with circulating leptin hormones, allowing them to transmit signals related to energy balance and metabolism.

Individuals with leptin receptor deficiency may have mutations or defects in these receptors that prevent them from properly recognizing and responding to leptin signals. This can lead to a decreased sensitivity to leptin and an imbalance in energy regulation, which can contribute to weight gain and other metabolic issues.

Leptin receptor deficiency can cause several health problems, including:

1. **Severe obesity**

    It is a major risk factor for several chronic diseases, including type 2 diabetes, cardiovascular disease, and certain types of cancer. Bariatric surgery is an effective treatment for severe obesity, but it is associated with a number of short- and long-term risks.

    Patients who undergo bariatric surgery are at risk for developing nutritional deficiencies due to the restrictions on food intake and the malabsorption of nutrients that can occur after surgery. These deficiencies can lead to a number of health problems, including anemia, osteoporosis, and impaired wound healing.

2. **High blood pressure**

    This is a condition in which the force of your blood against the walls of your arteries is high enough that it may eventually cause health problems, such as heart disease, stroke, or kidney issues. The increased workload on your heart can lead to the thickening of heart muscles and the narrowing of blood vessels over time.

High blood pressure usually doesn't have any symptoms, so you may not know that you have it. This is why it is often referred to as a "silent killer." Regular monitoring is crucial, as early detection can lead to effective management through lifestyle changes and medication. It's important to maintain a healthy diet, exercise regularly, and avoid excessive salt intake to help manage your blood pressure levels. Regular check-ups with your healthcare provider can help you stay on top of your health and catch any issues early.

3. **High cholesterol**

It is a waxy substance that's found in your blood. Having high cholesterol doesn't necessarily mean you have heart disease, but it's a risk factor.

High cholesterol is caused by a variety of things, including diet, genetics, and lifestyle. It can also be affected by other medical conditions, such as diabetes.

There are a couple of types of cholesterol: LDL and HDL. Considered the ***"bad" cholesterol is LDL***, which causes blockage by building up on the walls of your arteries. On the other hand, the ***"good" cholesterol is called HDL*** which helps remove LDL from your arteries.

4. **Type-2 diabetes**

   It is a chronic condition that affects your body's ability to use insulin properly. If you have type 2 diabetes, your body doesn't make enough insulin or doesn't use insulin well. Insulin assists in getting glucose into cells to give energy.

   Otherwise, glucose is retained in the blood if insulin is absent. If left untreated, high blood glucose may cause serious issues in the heart, kidneys, eyes, gums, teeth, and nerves.

   You can have type 2 diabetes at any age, even during childhood. However, this form of diabetes occurs most often in middle-aged and older people. Type 2 diabetes is also more common in people who are overweight or obese.

5. **Sleep apnea**

   This is a disorder where breathing stops temporarily a number of times the entire night. However, it is a common and treatable disorder. One of its initial signs is snoring loudly, but this doesn't mean everyone who snores loudly has sleep apnea. However, other symptoms include air gasping during sleep and daytime sleepiness.

   Sleep apnea can occur at any age, but it is most common in adults. It is more likely to occur if you are male, overweight, or have a family history of the condition.

Treating sleep apnea often improves your quality of life and may help prevent heart problems.

How Is Leptin Resistance Treated?

While there is no cure for leptin resistance, it can be effectively managed through diet and lifestyle changes. Here are several strategies to help manage leptin resistance:

- ***Eating Foods That Boost Leptin Sensitivity***: A healthy diet rich in fruits, vegetables, whole grains, lean proteins, and healthy fats can enhance leptin sensitivity. Nutrient-dense foods provide essential vitamins and minerals that support metabolic health and hormone balance.
- ***Avoiding Foods That Promote Leptin Resistance***: Limiting the intake of processed foods, sugary beverages, and unhealthy fats (such as those found in fried foods and certain snack items) is crucial. These foods can contribute to inflammation and metabolic disturbances, exacerbating leptin resistance.
- ***Exercising Regularly***: Physical activity is a powerful tool for increasing leptin sensitivity. Both aerobic exercises (like walking, running, and swimming) and strength training can improve overall metabolic

function, aid in weight management, and support hormonal health.

- *Maintaining a Healthy Weight*: Achieving and maintaining a healthy weight is essential in managing leptin resistance. Excess body fat, especially visceral fat, can impair leptin signaling. A balanced diet combined with regular exercise can help achieve sustainable weight loss and improve leptin responsiveness.
- *Managing Stress*: Chronic stress can negatively impact leptin sensitivity. Incorporating stress management techniques such as yoga, meditation, deep breathing exercises, and mindfulness can reduce stress levels and support hormonal balance.
- *Getting Adequate Sleep*: Quality sleep is critical for hormone regulation, including leptin. Ensuring sufficient and consistent sleep can help maintain proper leptin levels and improve overall metabolic health.
- *Hydration*: Staying well-hydrated is important for metabolic processes. Drinking plenty of water throughout the day helps regulate appetite and supports overall health.

By implementing these lifestyle changes, individuals can better manage leptin resistance, improve their metabolic health, and reduce the risk of associated conditions like obesity and type 2 diabetes. Consulting with healthcare professionals, such as dietitians or endocrinologists, can also provide personalized guidance and support.

Managing Leptin Resistance through Diet

Managing leptin resistance through diet involves making intentional food choices that optimize the body's sensitivity to leptin, a crucial hormone for regulating hunger and metabolism. By focusing on nutrient-dense, whole foods and maintaining regular eating patterns, you can enhance leptin function and support weight management efforts. This approach not only aims to balance hormone levels but also promotes overall health and well-being.

In this chapter, we will discuss the principles, benefits, and potential drawbacks of the leptin diet.

Principles of the Leptin Diet

The leptin diet is built around several key principles designed to enhance leptin sensitivity and improve overall health:

1. ***Eat Three Meals a Day***: Consume three balanced meals daily without snacking in between. This helps regulate natural hunger signals and supports leptin function, allowing your body to better manage energy

intake and expenditure. Make sure each meal includes a variety of nutrients to keep you feeling satisfied and energized throughout the day.
2. ***Stop Eating After Dinner***: Avoid eating for at least three hours before bedtime to give your body time to rest and reset overnight. This practice aids in digestion and can improve sleep quality, as your body is not working to process food while it's supposed to be resting and repairing.
3. ***Prioritize Protein***: Start each meal with a portion of high-quality protein to promote satiety and stabilize blood sugar levels. Proteins such as lean meats, beans, and tofu can help you feel fuller for longer, reducing the temptation to overeat or snack on unhealthy options between meals.
4. ***Avoid High-Sugar Foods***: Limit the intake of sugary and processed foods, as they can disrupt leptin sensitivity and lead to weight gain. High-sugar foods can cause spikes and crashes in blood sugar levels, making it harder to manage hunger and energy levels. Instead, opt for natural sources of sweetness like fruits.
5. *Incorporate Healthy Fats*: Include sources of healthy fats, such as avocados, nuts, and olive oil, which support hormone balance and overall health. These fats are essential for brain function, and cell regeneration, and can help reduce inflammation in the body. They

also play a crucial role in hormone production, which is vital for maintaining a balanced metabolism.

6. *Focus on Whole Foods*: Emphasize whole, unprocessed foods like vegetables, fruits, lean proteins, and whole grains to provide essential nutrients and maintain steady energy levels. Whole foods are rich in vitamins, minerals, and fiber, which are important for overall health and well-being. They help in maintaining a healthy gut microbiome, which is key to digestive health and immune function.

By adhering to these principles, you can support leptin function and work towards better health and weight management.

Benefits of The Leptin Diet

The leptin diet offers several benefits that can contribute to overall health and well-being:

1. *Improved Leptin Sensitivity*: By optimizing your body's response to leptin, the hormone that signals satiety, you can better regulate hunger and fullness. This improvement aids in maintaining a healthy weight by preventing overeating and supporting mindful eating habits.
2. *Weight Management*: The diet's emphasis on whole, nutrient-dense foods and structured eating times helps prevent overeating and supports sustainable weight

loss or maintenance. By focusing on natural, unprocessed foods, you are less likely to consume empty calories and more likely to stay full and satisfied.
3. ***Enhanced Metabolism***: Proper leptin function can boost your metabolism, helping your body efficiently convert food into energy. This increase in metabolic rate means you are burning more calories even at rest, which contributes to weight management and overall energy levels.
4. ***Stable Blood Sugar Levels***: Emphasizing proteins, healthy fats, and whole foods helps stabilize blood sugar levels, reducing the risk of insulin resistance and type 2 diabetes. Consistent blood sugar levels can also prevent the energy crashes and mood swings that are often associated with high-sugar diets.
5. ***Reduced Inflammation***: Avoiding processed foods and sugary snacks can lower inflammation in the body. Chronic inflammation is linked to various health issues, including heart disease, arthritis, and certain cancers. By reducing inflammation, you can potentially lower your risk of developing these chronic diseases.
6. ***Increased Energy Levels***: Balanced meals with adequate nutrients can lead to more consistent energy levels throughout the day. This can enhance overall productivity and vitality, allowing you to perform

better in daily activities and feel more alive and energetic.

7. ***Better Sleep Quality***: Following the principle of not eating close to bedtime can significantly improve sleep quality. Good sleep is essential for hormone regulation, cognitive function, and overall health. By ensuring you get a good night's sleep, you can improve your mood, concentration, and even physical health.

By focusing on these aspects, you can not only achieve a healthier body but also enjoy a better quality of life. Each of these benefits contributes to a holistic approach to wellness, where physical health, mental clarity, and emotional well-being are all interconnected.

Disadvantages of the Leptin Diet

While the leptin diet offers numerous health benefits, there are some disadvantages to consider:

1. ***Initial Adjustment Period***: Adapting to new meal patterns, especially cutting out snacks and late-night eating, can be challenging at first. It may take some time for your body to adjust to these changes. You might experience hunger pangs or cravings as your body acclimates, but these usually subside after a few weeks as you develop new eating habits.
2. ***Meal Planning Required***: The diet necessitates careful meal planning and preparation, which can be

time-consuming. Ensuring that each meal is balanced and nutrient-dense requires effort and dedication. This often involves researching recipes, grocery shopping for fresh ingredients, and cooking meals from scratch, which can be a significant shift for those used to eating out or relying on convenience foods.

3. *Avoidance of Processed Foods*: Eliminating sugary and processed foods from your diet can be difficult, particularly if you have strong cravings or are accustomed to convenience foods. Processed foods often contain added sugars, unhealthy fats, and preservatives that can be difficult to avoid. Transitioning to whole, unprocessed foods requires a mindful approach to eating and can also necessitate reading labels more carefully and making more informed choices.

4. *Social and Lifestyle Challenges*: Adhering to the diet may pose challenges during social gatherings or when dining out, as it can be harder to find compliant food options. You might find yourself needing to bring your own food to events or choosing restaurants with healthier options. Additionally, explaining your dietary choices to friends and family can sometimes be awkward or uncomfortable, especially if they do not share the same dietary habits.

Despite these disadvantages, the benefits of the leptin diet—such as improved leptin sensitivity, weight management, stable blood sugar levels, and enhanced overall health—far outweigh these initial hurdles. With commitment and consistency, the positive outcomes make the effort well worth it.

5 Step-by-Step Guide on How to Get Started with the Leptin Diet

It is important to note that before starting any new diet or lifestyle, it is best to consult with a healthcare professional. They can provide personalized recommendations and ensure that the diet is suitable for your individual needs. With that in mind, here is a step-by-step guide on how to get started with the leptin diet:

Step 1: Understand the Basics of Leptin

First, familiarize yourself with what leptin is and how it affects your body. Leptin is a hormone primarily produced by fat cells that plays a crucial role in regulating hunger and energy balance. Essentially, leptin serves as a communicator between your fat stores and your brain, signaling when you have enough energy stored and thus reducing appetite. When leptin levels are high, your brain receives the message that you are full, which helps to curb overeating. Conversely, low leptin levels signal hunger, prompting you to eat.

However, issues arise when the body becomes resistant to leptin, often due to an overconsumption of processed foods, sugar, and constant snacking, leading to a disrupted signaling process. This condition, known as leptin resistance, causes the brain to misinterpret leptin signals, resulting in persistent hunger and potential weight gain despite having adequate or excessive fat stores.

A leptin diet focuses on optimizing leptin sensitivity through mindful dietary choices and specific lifestyle changes. By prioritizing whole, unprocessed foods, establishing regular meal times, and incorporating healthy fats and proteins into your diet, you can enhance your body's response to leptin. Understanding these principles is the first step towards managing hunger more effectively, improving metabolic health, and ultimately achieving sustained weight management.

Step 2: Plan Your Meals

Creating a well-structured meal plan is a cornerstone of the leptin diet. A thoughtfully designed meal plan helps you keep your leptin levels in check, thereby promoting satiety and effective metabolism. Here's an in-depth look at the key points to focus on when planning your meals:

1. **Emphasize Whole, Unprocessed Foods**

    Choosing whole, unprocessed foods is essential for maintaining stable blood sugar levels and supporting leptin sensitivity. Nutrient-rich foods that are low in additives are more beneficial than their processed counterparts, which often lack essential vitamins and minerals while being high in unhealthy fats, sugars, and artificial ingredients.

Opt for fresh fruits and vegetables, whole grains, lean proteins, and healthy fats. These foods not only provide essential nutrients but also help stabilize blood sugar levels, preventing the spikes and crashes that can lead to leptin resistance.

2. **Incorporate High-Quality Proteins**

Protein is a vital component of any balanced diet, and it's particularly important for managing leptin levels. High-quality proteins promote feelings of fullness and maintain muscle mass, which in turn supports a healthy metabolic rate. Consider incorporating the following sources of protein into your meal plan:

- *Lean meats*: Options like chicken and turkey are excellent sources of protein without excessive saturated fat.
- *Fish*: Fatty fish such as salmon and tuna are rich in omega-3 fatty acids, which have anti-inflammatory properties and support brain health.

- *Eggs*: A versatile and nutrient-dense option, eggs provide high-quality protein along with essential vitamins and minerals.
- *Plant-based options*: Beans, lentils, and chickpeas are excellent sources of plant-based protein and fiber, making them great for those who prefer vegetarian or vegan diets.

3. **Include Healthy Fats**

    Healthy fats are crucial for hormone regulation, including leptin. They provide long-lasting energy and help you absorb fat-soluble vitamins (A, D, E, and K). Aim to include the following sources of healthy fats in your diet:

- *Avocados*: Rich in monounsaturated fats, avocados are also packed with fiber and various vitamins.
- *Nuts and seeds*: These are excellent sources of healthy fats, protein, and fiber. Almonds, walnuts, chia seeds, and flaxseeds are all great choices.
- *Olive oil*: Known for its heart-healthy monounsaturated fats, olive oil can be used for cooking or as a salad dressing.
- *Fatty fish*: In addition to being a protein source, fish like salmon and mackerel provide omega-3 fatty acids, which support overall health.

4. **Focus on Plenty of Vegetables**

   Vegetables are a powerhouse of nutrients and should form a substantial part of your meal plan. They are low in calories but high in vitamins, minerals, and fiber, contributing to satiety and overall health. Aim to include a variety of vegetables to cover a broad spectrum of nutrients:

- *Leafy greens*: Vegetables like spinach, kale, and Swiss chard are rich in vitamins A, C, and K, as well as iron and calcium.
- *Cruciferous vegetables*: Broccoli, cauliflower, and Brussels sprouts are known for their high fiber content and cancer-fighting compounds.
- *Root vegetables*: Carrots, sweet potatoes, and beets provide essential nutrients like beta-carotene, potassium, and fiber.

   Eating a colorful array of vegetables ensures you get a wide range of antioxidants and phytochemicals, which support overall health and well-being.

5. **Choose Complex Carbohydrates**

   Complex carbohydrates provide sustained energy and are less likely to cause blood sugar spikes compared to simple carbs. They are also rich in fiber, which aids digestion and promotes feelings of fullness. Some excellent choices for complex carbohydrates include:

- ***Whole grains***: Foods like quinoa, brown rice, and oats are high in fiber and nutrients. They provide a steady release of energy, keeping you full longer and helping regulate leptin levels.
- ***Legumes***: Beans, lentils, and peas are not only good sources of complex carbs but also provide protein and fiber.

6. **Avoid Sugary and Processed Foods**

   To maintain leptin sensitivity, it is crucial to avoid sugary and processed foods. These foods can cause rapid blood sugar spikes followed by crashes, leading to increased hunger and potential overeating. They can also interfere with leptin signals, making it harder for your brain to recognize when you're full.

Meal Planning Tips

1. ***Prepare meals in advance***: Batch cooking at the beginning of the week ensures you have healthy options readily available. This can prevent the temptation to reach for quick, unhealthy snacks during busy days.
2. ***Keep nutritious options on hand***: Stock your pantry and fridge with healthy staples like fresh vegetables, lean proteins, and whole grains. Having these items readily available makes it easier to stick to your dietary goals.

3. ***Plan balanced meals***: Ensure each meal includes a mix of protein, healthy fats, vegetables, and complex carbohydrates. This balance helps manage hunger levels and supports overall health.

By focusing on these key points, you can create a meal plan that enhances leptin sensitivity, supports weight management, and promotes overall health and well-being.

Step 3: Follow Structured Eating Times

Adhering to structured eating times is a crucial component of the leptin diet. By eating three balanced meals a day without snacking in between, you help your body maintain a natural rhythm that supports optimal leptin function. Here's how and why this works:

1. **Three Meals a Day:**
- ***Breakfast***: Start your day with a nutrient-dense breakfast that includes a balance of protein, healthy fats, and complex carbohydrates. This sets the tone for stable blood sugar levels and sustained energy throughout the morning.
- ***Lunch***: Midday, focus on a meal that continues to provide these essential nutrients, keeping you satiated and energized for the remainder of the day.
- ***Dinner***: Conclude your day with a lighter, balanced meal that ensures you're not overly full but still nourished.

2. **No Snacking Between Meals:**
- ***Regulates Hunger Signals***: Avoiding snacks helps your body rely on its natural hunger and fullness signals rather than constant external cues.
- ***Supports Leptin Sensitivity***: Frequent eating can lead to elevated insulin levels, which may interfere with leptin signaling. By sticking to three meals, you allow your hormones to function more efficiently.

3. **Timing of Dinner:**
- ***At Least Three Hours Before Bedtime***: Ensure that you finish dinner at least three hours before going to bed. This practice allows your body ample time to digest the food and reset overnight.
- ***Improves Sleep Quality***: Eating too close to bedtime can disrupt sleep, which is crucial for hormone regulation, including leptin.
- ***Metabolic Benefits***: Adequate time between your last meal and sleep can improve metabolic processes, promoting better fat utilization and overall health.

4. **Establishing a Routine:**
- ***Consistency is Key***: Try to have your meals at the same times each day. This consistency helps set your body's internal clock, making it easier to regulate hunger and satiety.
- ***Listen to Your Body***: Pay attention to your body's natural hunger cues. Over time, this structured eating

pattern can help you become more attuned to true hunger versus habitual or emotional eating.

Implementing structured eating times as part of your leptin diet not only aids in regulating leptin levels but also promotes a healthier relationship with food. By following these guidelines, you create a sustainable routine that supports long-term health and well-being.

Step 4: Incorporate Regular Exercise

Regular physical activity is a vital component of the leptin diet, playing a significant role in enhancing leptin sensitivity and promoting overall health. Here's how to effectively incorporate exercise into your routine:

1. **Support Leptin Sensitivity:**
- *Hormonal Balance*: Physical activity helps in regulating hormones, including leptin. It enhances the body's ability to respond to leptin signals, which can improve hunger regulation and energy balance.
- *Improved Insulin Sensitivity*: Exercise also boosts insulin sensitivity, reducing the risk of insulin resistance, which is often linked to leptin resistance.
2. **Recommended Exercise Duration and Intensity:**
- *At Least 30 Minutes of Moderate Exercise*: Aim for a minimum of 30 minutes of moderate-intensity exercise most days of the week. This duration is sufficient to

reap significant health benefits without causing excessive fatigue.

Examples of Moderate Exercise:

- *Brisk Walking*: A simple, accessible activity that elevates your heart rate and can be done almost anywhere.
- *Cycling*: Whether outdoors or on a stationary bike, cycling provides an excellent cardiovascular workout.
- *Swimming*: A low-impact exercise that works for multiple muscle groups and is gentle on the joints.
- *Dancing*: A fun way to get moving, improve coordination, and burn calories.

3. **Additional Exercise Options:**

- **Strength Training**: Incorporate weight lifting or bodyweight exercises (e.g., push-ups, squats) two to three times a week. Building muscle mass boosts metabolism and supports overall physical health.
- **Flexibility and Balance Exercises**: Activities like yoga or Pilates enhance flexibility, reduce injury risks, and promote mental well-being.

4. **Health Benefits Beyond Weight Management:**

- **Cardiovascular Health**: Regular exercise strengthens your heart, improves circulation, and reduces the risk of cardiovascular diseases.

- *Mental Health*: Physical activity releases endorphins, which can alleviate symptoms of depression and anxiety, improving overall mood.
- *Bone Density*: Weight-bearing exercises help maintain bone density, reducing the risk of osteoporosis.
- *Immune Function*: Engaging in regular exercise can boost your immune system, making you less susceptible to illnesses.

5. **Consistency and Enjoyment:**
- *Find Activities You Enjoy*: The best exercise is one that you enjoy and will stick with over the long term. Experiment with different activities to find what suits you best.
- *Make it a Habit*: Schedule exercise into your daily routine to ensure it becomes a consistent part of your lifestyle. Consistency is key to reaping the full benefits of physical activity.

Incorporating regular exercise into your leptin diet plan enhances leptin sensitivity, aids in weight management, and significantly improves overall health. By committing to at least 30 minutes of moderate exercise most days of the week, you set a strong foundation for a healthier, more active life.

Step 5: Monitor Your Progress

Monitoring your progress is a crucial step in the leptin diet journey, ensuring you stay committed and on track to achieve your health goals. Here's how to effectively keep tabs on your progress and make necessary adjustments:

1. **Track Your Meals:**
   - *Meal Logging*: Document what you eat at each meal, including portion sizes, ingredients, and any snacks or beverages. Regularly logging your meals helps you stay accountable, identify patterns or triggers, and make more mindful dietary choices. It can also be useful to note the time of day you eat and any feelings of hunger or fullness to better understand your eating habits.
   - *Nutrient Intake*: Pay close attention to the balance of proteins, fats, carbohydrates, vitamins, and minerals in your diet. Ensure you're meeting your nutritional needs while adhering to the principles of the leptin diet. This means not only counting macronutrients but also making sure you're getting a variety of fruits, vegetables, whole grains, and lean proteins to support overall health and well-being.

2. **Record Your Exercise Routines:**
   - *Workout Details*: Keep a detailed log of your workouts, noting the type of exercise, duration, intensity, and frequency. This helps you track your consistency and see tangible improvements over time. Additionally, it allows you to identify patterns and make necessary adjustments to your routine.

- *Variety and Progression*: Documenting your exercise routines allows you to incorporate variety and progressively challenge yourself. By doing so, you can prevent plateaus and maintain your motivation. This practice also ensures that you're not overworking the same muscle groups and are getting a well-rounded workout.

3. **Monitor How You Feel:**
- *Physical Well-being*: Track changes in energy levels, sleep quality, hunger signals, and overall physical health. These indicators can provide insights into how well your body is responding to the diet and exercise regimen. For instance, improved sleep quality can signify that your body is recovering efficiently, while increased energy levels may indicate better metabolic function and nutrient absorption.
- *Emotional and Mental Health*: Note any changes in mood, stress levels, and mental clarity. A well-balanced diet and regular exercise often lead to improved mental health and emotional stability. Additionally, regular physical activity can help release endorphins, which are known to boost mood and reduce feelings of anxiety and depression. Monitoring these aspects can help you recognize the positive impacts of your lifestyle changes on your overall well-being.

4. **Use Tools for Documentation:**
- *Journal*: A traditional journal is a simple and effective way to record your daily progress. Writing by hand can also be a reflective practice that helps you process your experiences. You can jot down your thoughts, feelings, and observations about your health journey, making it a personal and introspective activity that enhances self-awareness.
- *Apps and Digital Tools*: Numerous apps are available to track meals, exercise, and overall health. These tools can offer additional features such as calorie counting, nutrient analysis, and progress charts. Many apps also provide reminders, goal-setting functions, and community support, allowing you to stay motivated and connected with others on a similar health journey.

5. **Evaluate and Adjust:**
- *Regular Reviews*: Set aside dedicated time each week to thoroughly review your logs and assess your progress. Analyze your entries to look for patterns or areas where you might need to make adjustments. This could include noticing trends in your energy levels, mood, or physical performance.
- *Make Informed Changes*: If you notice certain foods or habits aren't serving you well, be proactive in making changes to improve your well-being. For example, if you find that late-night eating negatively affects your sleep quality, consider adjusting your

dinner timing or choosing lighter evening snacks. Making these informed changes can lead to significant improvements in your overall health and daily functioning.

6. **Celebrate Successes:**
- *Acknowledge Milestones*: Celebrate small victories along the way, whether it's sticking to your meal plan for a week, completing a challenging workout, or noticing improvements in how you feel. Recognizing these achievements can help sustain your motivation and remind you of the progress you are making, no matter how incremental.
- *Reward Yourself*: Consider non-food rewards such as a relaxing activity like a spa day, new workout gear like a pair of running shoes, or a fun outing such as a day trip to a local attraction. Positive reinforcement can significantly boost your motivation and help maintain long-term commitment to your fitness and wellness goals. Rewards provide a tangible way to acknowledge your hard work and encourage you to keep going.

By meticulously monitoring your meals, exercise routines, and overall well-being, you create a feedback loop that supports continuous improvement. This proactive approach ensures you remain engaged with your leptin diet journey, making it easier to optimize leptin levels and achieve your health goals.

Following these steps—understanding the basics of leptin, planning your meals, adhering to structured eating times, incorporating regular exercise, and monitoring your progress—you'll be well on your way to optimizing your leptin levels and achieving your health goals. Consistency, mindfulness, and a willingness to adjust as needed will support you in this endeavor, leading to lasting benefits for your overall well-being.

Foods to Eat

Incorporating certain foods into your diet can significantly enhance leptin sensitivity and support overall health. Here's a detailed look at some key nutritional components and the foods rich in them:

1. **Omega-3 Fatty Acids**

    Omega-3 fatty acids are known for their anti-inflammatory properties and their ability to improve leptin sensitivity. These essential fats are also crucial for maintaining heart health and preventing chronic diseases such as heart disease, stroke, and arthritis. Additionally, omega-3s can boost metabolism and aid in fat burning, making them beneficial for weight management.

    Foods rich in omega-3s include:

    - Salmon

- Mackerel
- Sardines
- Flaxseeds
- Chia seeds
- Walnuts
- Hemp seed
- Soybeans
- Eggs
- Spinach
- Kale
- Collard greens
- Brussels sprouts
- Cauliflower

2. **Fiber**

Fiber is a type of carbohydrate that is not absorbed by the body, which helps maintain satiety. Including fiber in your diet can assist with weight loss, relieve constipation, and regulate blood sugar levels. Fiber also promotes digestive health and has numerous other benefits.

High-fiber foods include:

- Beans (e.g., black beans, lentils)
- Legumes
- Whole grains (e.g., quinoa, oats)
- Vegetables

3. Antioxidants

Antioxidants protect cells from damage and have been associated with improved leptin sensitivity and increased thermogenesis. For example, green tea is high in antioxidants and has been shown to enhance leptin sensitivity and boost thermogenesis. Studies have found that green tea extract can increase levels of adiponectin, a hormone related to improved insulin sensitivity, and reduce pro-inflammatory cytokines.

Foods rich in antioxidants include:

- Green tea
- Dark chocolate
- Berries (e.g., blueberries, strawberries)
- Fruits (e.g., pomegranate, acai berry)

4. Healthy Fats

Healthy fats, such as those found in olive oil, avocados, and nuts, play a role in improving leptin sensitivity. These fats support overall health and help keep you feeling full longer, aiding in weight management.

Foods rich in healthy fats include:

- Olive oil
- Avocados
- Nuts (e.g., almonds, walnuts)

Significant Foods and Drinks for Leptin Sensitivity

Certain foods and beverages have been specifically linked to better leptin sensitivity due to their nutrient profiles and antioxidant content:

- *Green Tea*: Rich in antioxidants, it supports improved leptin sensitivity.
- *Oolong Tea*: A variety of green tea known to enhance leptin sensitivity.
- *Black Tea*: Contains antioxidants and is linked with better leptin sensitivity.
- *White Tea*: High in antioxidants and supportive of leptin sensitivity.
- *Herbal Teas*: Teas made from ginger or turmeric can help improve leptin sensitivity.
- *Fruit*: Especially berries, are rich in antioxidants that support leptin sensitivity.
- *Vegetables*: Particularly leafy greens are antioxidant-rich and support leptin sensitivity.
- *Whole Grains*: Such as quinoa and oats are high in fiber and aid in leptin sensitivity.
- *Beans*: Like black beans and lentils, they are fiber-rich and enhance leptin sensitivity.
- *Nuts*: Such as almonds and walnuts contain healthy fats that improve leptin sensitivity.

By integrating these foods into your diet, you can optimize leptin levels, support metabolic health, and work towards achieving your overall health goals.

Tips on How to Shop for Leptin Sensitivity-Boosting Foods

- *Choose Organic*: When possible, opt for organic fruits and vegetables to avoid potential pesticide residue that may interfere with leptin sensitivity.
- *Read Labels*: Be mindful of added sugars and unhealthy fats in packaged foods which can contribute to leptin resistance.
- *Shop Around the Perimeter*: Whole, fresh foods are typically found around the perimeter of the grocery store. Focus on filling your cart with these items rather than processed or packaged foods found in the center aisles.
- *Buy Frozen Foods*: Frozen fruits and vegetables can be just as nutritious as fresh ones and are often more affordable. Plus, they last longer so you can always have healthy options on hand.
- *Incorporate Variety*: Don't be afraid to try new foods and incorporate a variety of colors and textures into your diet. This will ensure you are getting a diverse range of nutrients to support leptin sensitivity.
- *Plan Ahead*: Make a list before heading to the grocery store and stick to it to avoid impulse purchases of

unhealthy foods. Also, consider meal prepping for the week ahead so that healthy options are easily accessible when hunger strikes.
- ***Shop at Farmers Markets***: Support local farmers and find fresh, seasonal produce at your local farmers market. This can also be a fun way to try new fruits and vegetables that may not be available in traditional grocery stores.

By following these tips, you can make healthier choices while shopping for foods that support leptin sensitivity. Remember, small changes over time can lead to big improvements in your overall health and well-being. Keep educating yourself on the importance of a balanced diet and stay disciplined with your food choices to support optimal leptin function.

Foods to Avoid

Certain foods can promote leptin resistance, making it more challenging for your body to effectively respond to this crucial hormone. Here are the main categories of foods you should avoid to support leptin sensitivity and overall health:

1. **Refined Carbohydrates**

    Refined carbohydrates are quickly absorbed, causing spikes in blood sugar levels. These spikes can lead to insulin resistance, affecting the body's response to leptin. Unlike unrefined carbs, refined ones lose their bran and germ during processing, reducing fiber and nutritional value. They also have a higher glycemic index, causing faster, significant rises in blood sugar.

Examples of refined carbs include:

- White flour
- White bread
- Pasta
- Cereal
- Sugar

2. **Trans Fats**

Trans fats are artificial fats created through partial hydrogenation, used by food manufacturers to increase shelf life and stabilize products. Found in many processed foods, they've been linked to insulin and leptin resistance. Trans fats raise bad cholesterol and lower good cholesterol, increasing the risk of heart disease and other health issues.

Foods high in trans fats include:

- Margarine
- Vegetable shortening
- Fried foods
- Processed baked goods
- Some processed foods

3. **Sugar**

   Sugar is a common ingredient in many sweet foods and drinks, offering a quick energy boost. However, too much sugar can cause inflammation, fat storage, and leptin resistance. It also leads to health problems like tooth decay, weight gain, and metabolic issues.

   Examples of sugary foods include:

- Candy
- Cookies
- Ice cream
- Pie
- Cake
- Bread
- Soda
- Fruit juice
- Sports drinks

4. **Alcohol**

   Alcohol can promote inflammation and fat storage, both of which can impair leptin sensitivity. Additionally, alcohol disrupts sleep patterns and acts as a diuretic, leading to dehydration. Poor sleep and dehydration can further contribute to weight gain and metabolic disturbances.

   Examples of alcoholic beverages include:

- Beer
- Wine
- Liquor
- Mixed drinks
- Cocktails

5. Processed Meats

Processed meats have been preserved through methods such as smoking, curing, and salting. These meats are typically high in salt and fat, which can lead to health issues if consumed in excess. Many processed meats also contain added nitrates and nitrites, chemicals linked to an increased risk of cancer.

Examples of processed meats include:

- Bacon
- Sausage
- Hot dogs
- Corned beef
- Ham
- Bologna

6. Soy Products

It is also advisable to avoid soy products. Although soy can be part of a healthy diet for some, certain people may experience adverse effects on hormone balance and leptin sensitivity.

Examples of soy products include:

- Soy sauce
- Tempeh
- Tofu
- Soybeans
- Soybean oils

By steering clear of these foods, you can help reduce the risk of developing leptin resistance and support a healthier, more balanced diet. This approach will aid in maintaining effective leptin signaling, contributing to better weight management and overall well-being.

Meal Plans to Add to Your Leptin-Resistance Diet

There are a few things you can do to make sure you're getting the most out of your leptin-resistance diet. First, be sure to eat breakfast within an hour of waking up.

Eating breakfast jump-starts your metabolism and helps to regulate your blood sugar levels throughout the day. It also provides your body with the energy it needs to get through the day.

Next, be sure to include protein at every meal. Protein helps to keep you feeling full and can help to reduce your overall calorie intake.

Finally, be sure to eat frequent meals throughout the day. Eating smaller meals more often can help regulate your blood sugar levels and keep your hunger under control.

Here are some meal ideas to get you started on your leptin-resistance diet:

Breakfast:

- 1 cup oatmeal with 1/2 cup berries and 1 scoop protein powder
- 2 eggs with 1 slice of whole-wheat toast and 1/2 avocado
- 1 smoothie made with 1 cup almond milk, 1 scoop protein powder, 1 cup spinach, and 1/2 banana

Lunch:

- 1 salad made with mixed greens, chicken, hard-boiled eggs, and avocado
- 1 bowl of soup made with lentils, kale, and carrots
- 1 turkey wrap made with whole wheat bread, lettuce, tomato, and avocado

Dinner:

- 1 salmon filet with roasted Brussels sprouts and sweet potato
- 1 chicken breast with sautéed kale and quinoa
- 1 veggie burger on a whole wheat bun with lettuce, tomato, and avocado

Snack:

- 1 apple with almond butter
- 1 cup plain Greek yogurt with berries
- 1 handful of nuts
- 1 hard-boiled egg

- 1 piece of fruit with cheese

A 7-Day Meal Plan

Below is a sample 7-day meal plan that you can either follow or modify, depending on your preference. Take note that you don't have to strictly prepare one recipe per meal. You can save leftovers and eat them for later.

	Breakfast	Lunch	Dinner
Day 1	Carrot Cake Oats	Tuna Salad	Fresh Cucumber Salad
Day 2	Green and Berry Smoothie	Creamy Low-FODMAP Fish Casserole	Greek Salad with Arugula
Day 3	Mediterranean Breakfast	Strawberry, Blueberry, and Spinach Salad	Chicken Breast with Herbs
Day 4	Healthy Green Smoothie	No-Fuss Tuna Casserole	Quinoa Lentil Salad
Day 5	No-Fuss Tuna Casserole	Quinoa Lentil Salad	Pecan and Maple Salmon
Day 6	Greek Salad with Arugula	Salmon with Sweet Potato and Kale	No-Fuss Tuna Casserole
Day 7	Mediterranean Breakfast	Chicken Breast with Herbs	Creamy Low-FODMAP Fish Casserole

Sample Recipes

We have also provided some sample recipes for you to try on your leptin-resistance diet. These recipes are all easy to prepare and incorporate the key principles of the diet – whole foods, protein, healthy fats, and low glycemic index carbohydrates.

Salmon with Sweet Potato and Kale

Ingredients:

- 1 lb. salmon
- 1 head of kale
- 1 sweet potato
- 1 tbsp. olive oil
- salt
- pepper

Instructions:

1. Preheat oven to 375°F.
2. Season salmon with salt and pepper.
3. Wash kale and chop it into bite-sized pieces.
4. Cut sweet potato into small cubes.
5. In a baking dish, place salmon in the center and surround it with kale and sweet potato.
6. Drizzle olive oil over everything and season with salt and pepper.
7. Bake for 20-25 minutes or until salmon is cooked through and vegetables are tender.
8. Serve immediately.

No-Fuss Tuna Casserole

Ingredients:

- 1-5 oz. can tuna, drained
- 1 can cream of chicken soup, condensed
- 3 cups macaroni, cooked
- 1-1/2 cups fried onions
- 1 cup Cheddar cheese, shredded

Instructions:

1. Preheat oven to 400°F.
2. In a large bowl, combine drained tuna, condensed soup, cooked macaroni, and half of the fried onions.
3. Transfer the mixture to a greased casserole dish.
4. Top with remaining fried onions and shredded cheese.
5. Bake for 20 minutes or until cheese is melted and bubbly.
6. Serve hot.

Pecan and Maple Salmon

Ingredients:

- 4 pcs. of 4 oz. salmon fillet
- 1/2 tsp. onion powder
- 1/2 tsp. chipotle pepper powder
- 1 tbsp. apple cider vinegar
- 1 tsp. smoked paprika
- 1/2 cup pecans
- salt
- ground black pepper
- 3 tbsp. pure maple syrup

Instructions:

1. Preheat oven to 375°F.
2. In a small bowl, mix onion powder, chipotle pepper powder, apple cider vinegar, and smoked paprika.
3. Season salmon fillets with salt and black pepper on both sides.
4. Spread the mixture evenly over each salmon fillet.
5. Crush pecans into small pieces and press onto the top of each salmon fillet.
6. Drizzle maple syrup over the pecan-coated salmon.
7. Bake for 15-20 minutes or until fish is cooked through and flaky.
8. Serve hot with your choice of side dish.

Velvety Herbed Pumpkin

Ingredients:

- 3 cups of pumpkin, skin removed and flesh cut roughly into half-inch cubes
- 1 medium onion, chopped finely
- 3 garlic cloves, minced
- 2 serrano or jalapeno chilies, chopped finely (use less if you like less heat or take out the seeds and ribs)
- 7-8 medium-sized sage leaves, minced
- 2 tbsp. cilantro or coriander leaves, chopped finely
- 2 tsp. sugar
- 1 tbsp. canola or other vegetable oil
- salt, to taste

Instructions:

1. In a large pot, heat oil over medium-high heat.
2. Add onions and garlic, and cook until translucent.
3. Add chilies and sage leaves, and stir well for 1-2 minutes.
4. Stir in pumpkin cubes, sugar, and salt. Allow to cook for 10-15 minutes or until pumpkin is tender.
5. Once cooked through, turn off the heat and add chopped cilantro or coriander leaves on top.

6. Let it cool for a few minutes before blending until smooth (you can use an immersion blender or transfer to a regular blender).
7. Serve hot with your choice of bread or crackers on the side.

Greek Salad with Arugula

Ingredients:

- 1-1/2 lbs. or 750 g sweet potatoes, washed well
- salt, preferably Greek sea salt
- 1 large red onion or a bunch of scallions, sliced thinly
- 2 bunches of fresh arugula, coarsely chopped
- 1/2 virgin Greek olive oil
- 3-4 tbsp. red wine vinegar

Instructions:

1. Preheat the oven to 400°F.
2. Peel and cut sweet potatoes into bite-sized cubes.
3. On a baking sheet, arrange the sweet potato cubes in a single layer.
4. Sprinkle with salt and drizzle with olive oil.
5. Roast for about 25-30 minutes or until they are nice and browned on the outside.
6. Meanwhile, in a large mixing bowl, toss together red onion or scallions and arugula leaves.
7. In a small bowl, mix olive oil and red wine vinegar to make the dressing.
8. Once roasted sweet potatoes have cooled down slightly, add them to the salad mixture.

9. Pour dressing over the top of the salad and gently toss everything together until well combined.
10. Serve immediately as a side dish or add grilled chicken or shrimp to make it a complete meal.

Tuna Salad

Ingredients:

- 1/2 cup pecans
- 1 cup chicken breast, steamed and cubed
- 1 cup tuna in oil
- salt, to taste
- pepper, to taste

Instructions:

1. In a dry skillet, toast pecans over medium heat for about 5 minutes, stirring frequently.
2. Remove from heat and let them cool before chopping them coarsely.
3. In a mixing bowl, combine chicken breast and tuna with salt and pepper to taste.
4. Top with chopped toasted pecans.
5. Serve on top of a bed of greens or in your choice of bread or crackers for a tasty sandwich or wrap option.

Chicken Breast with Herbs

Ingredients:

- 1 tsp. dried oregano
- 1/2 tsp. rosemary
- 1/2 tsp. garlic powder
- 1/8 tsp. teaspoon salt
- black pepper, finely ground
- 4 chicken breasts

Instructions:

1. Preheat oven to 375°F.
2. In a small bowl, mix oregano, rosemary, garlic powder, salt, and pepper.
3. Rub the herb mixture onto both sides of the chicken breasts.
4. Place the chicken in a baking dish and bake for 25-30 minutes or until internal temperature reaches 165°F.
5. Let it rest for 5 minutes before slicing and serving.

Creamy Low-FODMAP Fish Casserole

Ingredients:

- 1-1/2 lb. white fish, serving-sized pieces
- 2 tbsp. olive oil
- 2 tbsp. small capers
- 1 lb. broccoli
- 1 oz. grass-fed butter
- 6 scallions
- 1 tbsp. Dijon mustard
- 1 tbsp. dried barley
- 1 tsp. salt
- 1/4 tsp. ground black pepper*

Instructions:

1. Preheat oven to 375°F.
2. In a large baking dish, lay fish pieces in one layer and drizzle with olive oil.
3. Sprinkle capers over the fish and bake for 10 minutes or until flaky.
4. While the fish is cooking, steam broccoli until soft but not mushy and set aside.
5. In a small saucepan, melt butter over low heat and add chopped scallions, mustard, barley, salt, and pepper.
6. Cook on low heat for about 1-2 minutes until the mixture thickens.

7. Pour sauce over the fish and top with steamed broccoli before returning to the oven for an additional 10 minutes.
8. Serve hot as a main dish with your choice of side dishes.

*black pepper may be substituted with white pepper

Green and Berry Smoothie

Ingredients:

- 2 cups spinach
- 2 large kale leaves
- 3/4 cup water
- 1 large frozen banana
- 1/2 cup frozen mango
- 1/2 cup frozen peach
- 1 tbsp. ground flaxseeds
- 1 tbsp. almond butter or peanut butter

Instructions:

1. In a blender, combine spinach, kale, water, and ground flaxseeds.
2. Blend until smooth, scraping down the sides if needed.
3. Add frozen banana, mango, peach, and nut butter to the blender and blend again until well combined.
4. If the texture is too thick for your liking, add more water as needed to reach desired consistency.

Optional: top with fresh berries or additional toppings of your choice before serving.

Healthy Green Smoothie

Ingredients:

- 1 cup fresh spinach
- 1/2 tsp. mint extract or to taste
- Optional: 1/4 tsp. peppermint liquid Stevia

Instructions:

1. In a blender, combine spinach and mint extract.
2. Blend until smooth, scraping down the sides if needed.
3. Optional: add liquid Stevia for added sweetness and blend again until well combined.
4. Serve immediately or store in an airtight container in the fridge for up to 24 hours.

Mediterranean Breakfast

Ingredients:

- 2 eggs, either poached or hard-boiled
- 1/2 medium avocado, diced
- 1 cup tomato, diced
- 1 cup cucumber, diced
- parsley, chopped, for garnish

Instructions:

1. In a bowl or on a plate, arrange the poached or hard-boiled eggs.
2. Top with diced avocado, tomato, cucumber, and parsley.
3. Serve with whole-grain toast for a complete breakfast.

Optional: add a sprinkle of feta cheese or a drizzle of olive oil for added flavor.

Carrot Cake Oats

Ingredients:

- 1/2 cup dry oats, cooked in water
- 1 scoop vanilla whey protein powder
- 3 oz. unsweetened almond milk
- 2-3 tbsp. carrots, grated
- allspice, to taste
- cinnamon, to taste
- nutmeg, to taste
- 1 tbsp. maple syrup
- Optional: 1 tbsp. sliced almonds
- Optional: 1 tbsp. shaved coconut

Instructions:

1. In a medium saucepan, cook oats according to package instructions using water.
2. Once cooked, stir in protein powder and unsweetened almond milk until well combined.
3. Add grated carrots and spices (allspice, cinnamon, nutmeg) to taste.
4. Continue cooking for an additional 2-3 minutes.
5. Serve hot and drizzle with maple syrup.

Optional: top with sliced almonds and/or shaved coconut for added texture and flavor.

Fresh Cucumber Salad

Ingredients:

- 1 English cucumber, large, halved and sliced
- 2 cups grape tomatoes, halved
- 1 red onion, medium, sliced thinly
- 1/2 cup balsamic vinaigrette
- 3/4 cup reduced-fat feta cheese, crumbled

Instructions:

1. In a large bowl, combine sliced cucumber, halved grape tomatoes, and thinly sliced red onion.
2. Pour balsamic vinaigrette over the vegetables and toss to coat evenly.
3. Sprinkle crumbled feta cheese on top and gently mix in with the vegetables.
4. Serve as a refreshing side dish or add grilled chicken or chickpeas for a protein-packed meal.

Quinoa Lentil Salad

Ingredients:

- 2/3 cups dried brown lentils
- 2 cups water
- 1 cup quinoa
- 1 yellow sweet pepper, diced
- 1 shallot, chopped
- 1 bunch of arugula, finely chopped
- 2 tsp. Dijon mustard
- 1/4 cup lemon juice
- 1/4 cup extra virgin olive oil
- 1/3 cup crumbled feta cheese
- 1 pinch salt
- 4 tbsp. fresh mint, chopped

Instructions:

1. In a medium pot, bring 2 cups of water to a boil.
2. Rinse the lentils and add them to the boiling water. Reduce heat and simmer for about 20 minutes or until lentils are tender.
3. While the lentils are cooking, rinse the quinoa in a fine-mesh strainer and cook according to package instructions using water.
4. Once both lentils and quinoa are cooked, let them cool for 10-15 minutes.

5. In a large bowl, combine diced yellow pepper, chopped shallot, and finely chopped arugula with the cooled lentils and quinoa.
6. In a separate small bowl, whisk together Dijon mustard, lemon juice, extra virgin olive oil, and a pinch of salt to make the dressing.
7. Pour the dressing over the lentil and quinoa mixture and toss to coat evenly.
8. Top with crumbled feta cheese and chopped fresh mint for added flavor.
9. Serve as a hearty lunch or dinner option, or add grilled shrimp or tofu for an extra boost of protein.

Strawberry, Blueberry, and Spinach Salad

Ingredients:

- 5 strawberries, chopped
- 10 blueberries, chopped
- 1-1/2 cups baby spinach
- 1 oz. crumbled goat cheese
- 4 walnuts, crushed

For the salad dressing:

- 1/2 tbsp. extra-virgin olive oil
- cracked black pepper
- 1/2 tbsp. rice wine vinegar

Instructions:

1. In a large mixing bowl, combine chopped strawberries and blueberries with baby spinach leaves.
2. Add crumbled goat cheese and crushed walnuts to the mixture.
3. In a small bowl, whisk together extra-virgin olive oil, cracked black pepper, and rice wine vinegar to create a simple dressing.
4. Drizzle the dressing over the salad mixture and toss to coat evenly.
5. Serve as a refreshing side dish or add grilled chicken for a complete meal.

Conclusion

Thank you for sticking with us to the end of this comprehensive guide on managing leptin through diet. Your commitment to understanding how leptin influences your body and how you can manage it through food choices is commendable. This dedication speaks volumes about your desire to improve your health and well-being.

Leptin, as we've explored, is a hormone that plays a pivotal role in regulating both your appetite and metabolism. When leptin functions as it should, it helps you maintain a healthy weight and reduces the risk of obesity-related conditions. Unfortunately, when leptin signaling is impaired, it can lead to overeating and weight gain, creating a challenging cycle to break. The encouraging news is that you have the power to positively impact your leptin levels with thoughtful dietary and lifestyle choices.

As you move forward, remember that small, consistent changes can make a substantial difference in your journey toward better leptin management. Incorporating whole foods such as vegetables, fruits, lean proteins, and healthy fats into your daily meals can significantly improve your leptin sensitivity. Steering clear of processed foods and sugary snacks will not only benefit your waistline but also support your body's natural hormone balance.

You're not alone in facing these challenges. Many people struggle with leptin resistance, but with dedication and the right approach, you can overcome it. Focus on the quality of your food rather than just the quantity. Eating mindfully, paying attention to your body's hunger signals, and avoiding emotional eating are all strategies that can help you regain control over your appetite.

Exercise is another powerful ally in managing leptin. Regular physical activity enhances leptin sensitivity and helps regulate your appetite. Whether it's going for a brisk walk, practicing yoga, or engaging in more intense workouts, find something you enjoy and make it part of your routine. Exercise doesn't have to be a chore; it can be an enjoyable way to boost your mood, energy levels, and overall health.

Sleep is equally vital. Lack of sleep can disrupt your hormone levels, including leptin, leading to increased hunger and cravings. Prioritize good sleep hygiene by setting a regular sleep schedule, creating a restful environment, and avoiding stimulants like caffeine before bedtime. Quality sleep can significantly impact both your weight management efforts and overall well-being.

Staying hydrated is often overlooked but crucial for leptin management. Sometimes thirst is mistaken for hunger, which can lead to unnecessary snacking. Drinking plenty of water throughout the day keeps you hydrated and helps regulate your appetite.

Stress management also plays a crucial role. Chronic stress can lead to hormonal imbalances, including leptin resistance. Finding ways to manage stress—such as through meditation, relaxation techniques, or hobbies you enjoy—can positively impact your leptin levels and overall health.

As you implement these changes, be patient with yourself. Hormonal balance takes time, and progress may be slow at first. Celebrate small victories along the way and stay motivated by focusing on how these changes make you feel, rather than just the numbers on the scale.

Your journey toward better leptin management and overall health is unique. Listen to your body, make adjustments as needed, and be open to learning and experimenting with different strategies. What works for one person might not work for another, and that's okay. The key is to find what works best for you and stick with it.

By taking control of your diet, exercise, sleep, hydration, and stress levels, you're setting yourself up for long-term success. These lifestyle changes are not just about managing leptin; they're about creating a healthier, happier you. Embrace the journey and give yourself credit for the positive steps you're taking.

Thank you again for reading this guide. We hope you found it informative and empowering. Remember, every step you take towards better leptin management is a step towards a healthier life. Keep going, stay informed, and most importantly, believe in yourself. You have the tools and knowledge to make meaningful changes. Now, it's time to put them into action.

Stay committed, stay positive, and watch as your efforts pay off in improved health and well-being. You've got this!

FAQs

What is leptin?

Leptin is a hormone that plays a role in energy balance and metabolism.

What is leptin resistance?

Leptin resistance is a condition in which the body does not respond properly to leptin's signals. This can lead to overeating and weight gain.

What are some foods that can help to improve leptin sensitivity?

Foods that can help to improve leptin sensitivity include omega-3 fatty acids, fiber, antioxidants, and healthy fats.

What are some lifestyle changes that can help to manage leptin resistance?

Lifestyle changes that can help to manage leptin resistance include getting regular exercise, sleeping 7-8 hours per night, and managing stress.

Can leptin resistance be reversed?

There is no cure for leptin resistance, but it is possible to manage it with diet and lifestyle changes.

Helpful Questions Regarding Leptin Resistance

What if my leptin level is high?

If your leptin level is high, it may be due to obesity or another medical condition. If you are obese, you may be able to improve your leptin levels with weight loss. If you have a medical condition, you should talk to your doctor about treatment options.

What if my leptin level is low?

If your leptin level is low, it may be due to malnutrition or another medical condition. If you are malnourished, you may be able to improve your leptin levels with proper nutrition. If you have a medical condition, you should talk to your doctor about treatment options.

What is the difference between leptin and ghrelin?

Leptin and ghrelin are two hormones that play a role in energy balance. Leptin is produced by fat cells and signals to the brain that the body has enough energy. Ghrelin is produced by the stomach and signals to the brain that the body needs more energy.

What are some other hormones involved in energy balance?

Other hormones involved in energy balance include insulin, glucagon, and cortisol.

What are some other ways to increase leptin sensitivity?

In addition to diet and lifestyle changes, there are some supplements that may help to increase leptin sensitivity. These include omega-3 fatty acids, fiber, antioxidants, and healthy fats. You should talk to your doctor before taking any supplements.

What are the long-term effects of leptin resistance?

Leptin resistance can lead to weight gain and obesity. Obesity is a risk factor for many chronic diseases, such as heart disease, diabetes, and cancer. Therefore, it is important to manage leptin resistance to reduce your risk of these diseases.

What if I suspect that I have leptin resistance?

If you think you may have leptin resistance, you should talk to your doctor. They can order tests to check your leptin levels and determine if you have any underlying medical conditions. They can also provide guidance on how to manage leptin resistance with diet and lifestyle changes.

References and Helpful Links

Types of fat. (2024, May 9). The Nutrition Source. https://nutritionsource.hsph.harvard.edu/what-should-you-eat/fats-and-cholesterol/types-of-fat/

Professional, C. C. M. (n.d.-d). Leptin & Leptin Resistance. Cleveland Clinic. https://my.clevelandclinic.org/health/articles/22446-leptin

Sachithanandan, A. (2013). eComment. Paradigm shift in surgery for massive pulmonary embolism: If not now then when? Interactive Cardiovascular and Thoracic Surgery, 17(2), 246. https://doi.org/10.1093/icvts/ivt274

Leptin Resistance Diet: A beginner's 3-Step plan to managing leptin resistance through diet, with sample recipes and a 7-Day meal plan : Gilta, Brandon: Amazon.com.au: Books. (n.d.). https://www.amazon.com.au/Leptin-Resistance-Diet-Beginners-Managing/dp/B0B86PB8BD

Andreotti, G., Koutros, S., Hofmann, J. N., Sandler, D. P., Lubin, J. H., Lynch, C. F., Lerro, C. C., De Roos, A. J., Parks, C. G., Alavanja, M. C., Silverman, D. T., & Freeman, L. E. B. (2017). Glyphosate use and cancer incidence in the Agricultural Health study. Journal of the National Cancer Institute, 110(5), 509–516. https://doi.org/10.1093/jnci/djx233

Wiginton, K. (2023, February 14). Foods to boost leptin? WebMD. https://www.webmd.com/diet/foods-to-boost-leptin

Liu, J., Yang, X., Yu, S., & Zheng, R. (2018). The leptin resistance. In Advances in experimental medicine and biology (pp. 145–163). https://doi.org/10.1007/978-981-13-1286-1_8

www.ingramcontent.com/pod-product-compliance
Lightning Source LLC
LaVergne TN
LVHW010411070526
838199LV00065B/5946